I HAVE A FRIEND
WHO IS BLIND

HANNAH CARLSON, M.ED, CRC
DALE CARLSON

illustrated by
HOPE M. DOUGLAS, M.A.

CHANEY SHANNON PRESS
BICK PUBLISHING HOUSE

MADISON, CT

Edited by Ann Maurer

With thanks to Alan Ecker, M.D., Assistant Clinical Professor of
Opthalmology at Yale University

CHANEY SHANNON PRESS is a trademark of
BICK PUBLISHING HOUSE

Library of Congress Catalog Card Number: 95-79842

ISBN: 1-884158-07-2 –Volume 2
ISBN: 1-884158-11-0 -- 4 Volume Set

Printed by Royal Printing Service, Guilford, USA

Special needs/disabilities

"These books are an important service. They are informed, practical guides to feelings, behavior patterns, medical facts, technology, and resources for people who care about people with disabilities."
    –Richard Fucci, former president of the National Spinal
      Cord Injury Association

"Excellent, very informative."
    –Alan R. Ecker, M.D., Assistant Clinical Professor of
      Opthalmology, Yale University

"An invaluable source of help and comfort for friends and caregivers of people who have disabilities or special needs."
    –Mary Jon Edwards, Nationally Certified Therapeutic
      Horseback Riding Instructor, Special Olympics

"Excellent introductory handbooks about disabilities and special needs. They discuss medical conditions and rehabilitation, feelings and adaptive technology, and responsible attitudes both on the part of people with disabilities and people temporarily without them. The emphasis is on our common humanity, not our differences."
    –Lynn McCrystal, M.ED.,vice-president, The Kennedy Center

"The books offer professional information in an easy-to-use, uncomplicated style."
    –Renee Abbott, Group Home Director, S.A.R.A.H.,
      Shoreline Association for the Retarded and Handicapped

"Precise information, good reading for the layperson."
    –Jane Chamberlin, parent and employment supervisor, West
      Haven Community House

"Thank you for the opportunity to be a part of this work."
    –Christine M. Gaglio, employment specialist for the deaf, The
      Kennedy Center

CONTENTS

NOTE

The real problems of blindness are not necessarily the loss of eyesight. The real problems are our misinformed or discourteous attitudes. Blindness does not discriminate. Any baby can be born blind; any adult can become blind. If a blind person has training and opportunity, blindness is not a tragedy in helplessness, it is mostly a physical nuisance.

People who are blind are usually portrayed in two ways: those who are totally helpless and can't do anything; and those who are superhuman and can do everything. The truth is that people who are blind or visually impaired can do most things and need help with some things.

If you are family or caregiver, old friend, new acquaintance, or stranger on a bus, it's good to learn that it is hard to be blind in a world so insistant on visual cues, and on regarding a physical limitation as a kind of failure.

In a world that tends to avoid or misunderstand, an intelligent and informed offer of help and a knowledge of the resources available are a godsend to us all.

ACKNOWLEDGMENTS

Our gratitude to Theodore Harold Bromm and Renee Abbott, Group Home Director, both of S.A.R.A.H., the Shoreline Association of the Retarded and Handicapped; to Richard Fucci, former president of the National Spinal Cord Injury Association; to Alan Ecker, M.D., Assistant Clinical Professor of Opthalmolgy at Yale University; to Jane Chamberlin, parent and employment supervisor, West Haven Community House; and to Lynn McCrystal, M.Ed., vice-president, The Kennedy Center, for their counsel and editorial advice.

Our gratitude to Louis and Susan Weady, not only for Royal Printing, but for their guidance and patience with new editions, purchase orders, and shipping.

Our special thanks to Herb Swartz for his kindness and the use of his computers.

Our further special thanks to Danny Carlson for teaching us how to use computer capabilities for publishing.

And our thanks to Terrence Finnegan for providing Bick Publishing House with its own computer system.

5

1

CAUSES AND CONDITIONS OF BLINDNESS

People can be blind at birth. They can go blind slowly, or swiftly, traumatically. Age, circumstances, and disposition affect each blind person differently. But living in a sighted world in a sighted culture, with sighted ambitions and dreams and pleasures, sighted tempo and obstructions, sighted communications and attitudes about independence is always staggeringly difficult, sometimes despairingly lonely. Just the necessity of having to live life more slowly and deliberately in a fast and careless world can be a daily frustration.

Visual impairment and blindness

• An individual is visually impaired if the best corrected distant visual acuity in the better eye is 20/80 or less, or if visual

E	20/200
	20/100
F P	20/70
T O Z	20/50
L P E D	20/40
P E C F D	20/30
E D F C Z P	20/25
F E L O P E D D E F P O T E C	20/20

fields are significantly restricted (visual acuity is expressed as a fraction – the test distance, 20 feet, over the figure assigned to the lowest line the person can read).

• Just being nearsighted or farsighted, having focused problems(astigmatism), can normally be adjusted with corrective lenses and do not lead to blindness.

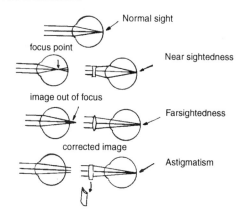

Normal sight

focus point

Near sightedness

image out of focus

Farsightedness

corrected image

Astigmatism

• Legal blindness (partial) in the USA is defined as visual acuity for distant vision of 20/200 or less in the better eye with best correction, or if the visual field is reduced to a diameter of 20 degrees or less (such as severe loss of peripheral vision).

• There are about 1,000,000 legally blind people in the USA, about 1/2 of whom are over 65. Major causes are: glaucoma; diabetic retinopathy; and macular degeneration.

• There are an estimated 28 million people worldwide who have eyesight of 10/200 or less, and millions more have loss of sight sufficient to interfere with normal living. Major causes worldwide are: cataract, trachoma (contagious conjunctivitis), leprosy, onchocerciasis (infestation of worms transmitted by blackfly), conjunctival dryness due to lack of vitamin A.

The categories of blindness include:

Trauma

Genetic disorders, birth defects and injury

Chronic, acute, and infectious diseases of the eye or involving vision

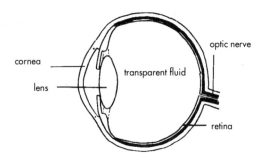

TRAUMA

Injuries: automobile accidents, military combat, criminal (beatings, gunshot, battering, abuse), sports, workplace (explosions, fires, foreign bodies), even the bizarre accidents of ordinary life, are significant causes of blindness.

Foreign bodies: danger of infection, resultant ulcer of the cornea, sympathetic opthalmia (transference of inflammation from an injury of one eye to the normal eye; loss of vision in both eyes may result).

Corneal abrasion: injury to the eye involving fingernail, piece of paper, contact lens, and so forth.

Contusions: "black eye," may cause hemorrhage, swelling, rupture of the cornea, cataract, tears and detachment of the retina, fracture of the orbital floor (the bony cavity of the skull that contains and protects the eyeball), glaucoma, cut or injured optic nerves.

Lacerations: of the lids or mucous membranes that line the lid (conjunctiva) or the cornea.

Ultraviolet burns: from sunlamps, skiing, exposure to welding arc without protection.

Chemical burns: cause scarring, adhesions, tear duct obstruction, secondary infection.

GENETIC DISORDERS, BIRTH DEFECTS AND INJURY
Genetic Disorders

Chromosomes are the vehicles in which the genes are carried from generation to generation. Virtually all characteristics, and this includes diseases as well as human traits such as personality, height, and intelligence, are to some extent determined by the genes.

Genetic changes, alterations, and disorders are termed mutations. These can be inherited or spontaneous, and can produce congenital anomalies.

Absence of eyes or functioning parts.

Defects of structures such as: failure of eyelids to separate; refractive errors such as progressive myopia; congenital nystagmus (wandering eyes associated with absence of central vision);

drooping upper eyelid from paralysis; third nerve palsy; congenital cataracts; congenital glaucoma.

Diseases such as retinitis pigmentosa. This is a hereditary, chronic, progressive disease characterized by the degeneration of the retina, atrophy of the optic nerve, pigmentary changes in the retina. In childhood symptoms begin, such as defective night vision, followed by constrictions in the field of vision. So far, there is no cure.

Birth Defects and Injury

Genetic disorders are often referred to as birth defects, but there are also groups of conditions arising either from the birth process itself, or the mother's health and condition during pregnancy. Any of these may cause blindness.

Infections in mother:
Congenital toxoplasmosis (infection of central nervous system caused by protozoa sometimes caught from animal feces)
Syphilis

Strangling umbilical cord: if the brain is deprived of oxygen for too long, there may be developmental defects.

Drugs: the mother's ingestion of improper drugs can affect proper development of the fetus.

10

Improper nutrition and prenatal care

Conditions in the mother's health, such as rubella, HIV, or AIDS, can produce lifelong vision disabilities in the child.

Improper care and conditions at the time of delivery can affect a baby's eyesight. Blindness occurs if premature infants are exposed to too high a concentration of oxygen as part of their therapy, as happened to Stevie Wonder.

CHRONIC, ACUTE, AND INFECTIOUS DISEASES OF THE EYE OR INVOLVING VISION

Leading causes of blindness

Glaucoma

This is a disease of the eye characterized by the pressure of fluid that cannot drain properly out of the eye. The pressure builds up in the eye against the optic nerve and damages this important nerve that connects the eye to the brain. The result is atrophy of the optic nerve and blindness. There are two types: in acute glaucoma, there is rapid onset, severe pain, and profound visual loss, red eye, steamy cornea, the complaint of lights with halos. Untreated, blindness can result in days. The second type of glaucoma is usually slow in onset and painless, and can be treated successfully in the early stages with medication, and sometimes surgery. Without a specialist, Ray Charles was blind from glaucoma by the age of seven.

Diabetic Retinopathy

This disorder of the retina in someone with diabetes causes blindness. Diabetes affects the blood sugar levels; blood sugar levels affect the blood vessels in the retina. The blood vessels break and bleed into the clear fluid in the eye, blurring vision. Scar tissue forms that may pull the retina away from the coat of the eye and cause retinal detachment.

Macular Degeneration

This is a breakdown of sight in the retina, the leading cause of permanent visual loss of central vision, though not necessarily peripheral vision, in the elderly. The exact cause is unknown. There is no specific treatment, but there are low vision aids.

Cataract

A cataract is a lens opacity, a clouding of the lens of the eye. Blurred vision is progresssive over the years. There is no pain or redness with cataracts. Cataracts may be congenital (owing to mother contracting rubella, for instance). There may be genetic errors of metabolism or other hereditary factors. They may be caused by trauma, or secondary to systemic disease, or associated with uveitis. Senile cataract is the most common; it occurs among persons over the age of sixty. The cloudy lens is removed by surgery, and an intraocular lens implanted. The rate of success is 95% (Keep the head above the heart after eye surgery!)

Other diseases and disorders of the eye

Retinoblastoma: cancer of the retina, more often in the young
Tumors of the eye and lid, benign and malign
Conjunctivitis: the most common eye disease.   Conjunctivitis can
be acute or chronic; it can be caused by bacterial or viral infection, even allergies that are severe enough to cause blindness.
Trachoma is the most serious of its forms.
Optic neuritis: inflammation due to a variety of diseases ranging
from multiple sclerosis to viral infections such as mumps.
AIDS: many possible complications involving the eye; cotton
wool spots, retinal spathces, hemorrhages, optic nerve problems,
retinal detachment, herpes simplex and zoster infections, toxo-
plasmic infections.

Some eye disorders are genetic or not yet curable. Many are
curable or can be arrested if treated early and expertly.

But any change in vision in anyone, regardless of whether
the change is related to a chronic condition or occurs suddenly,
requires an immediate consultation with an opthalmologist or a
general practitioner. You may prefer to escort your friend or relative with the vision problem to the nearest eye clinic, even an
emergency clinic. But do not allow any change in vision in anyone to go unattended to or unexamined.   Immediate attention
can make the difference, if a difference can be made, in the
degree to which vision is affected.

But if blindness has to be, let people think of it in the way
John Hull, professor of religious philosophy and author of

13

Touching the Rock, An Experience of Blindness , describes. He began to think of himself not "as lacking something, but simply as a whole-body-seer...simply someone in whom the specialized function of sight is now devolved upon the whole body, and no longer specialized in a particular organ...it is a state, like the state of being young, or of being old, of being male or female; it is one of the orders of human being."

2

THEIR FEELINGS, YOUR FEELINGS

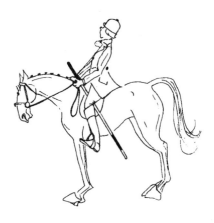

There is a woman who lost her sight to glaucoma when she was less than thirty. When offered a riding class for the disabled, her answer was: "I'm not disabled. I can ride a horse. I just can't see."

Ray Charles, the first to play what is called "soul," recalls that when he went blind at the age of seven, his mother said, "You're blind, not stupid. You've lost your eyes, not your mind."

In the journals and books written by people who are blind about their blindness, what is said frequently is that among the greatest losses is the communication of the eyes, eye meeting eye with love or lust, humor, the unspoken word. What is gained, because it is simply impossible to hurry, is time. Space no longer exists, or shrinks. But there is slowed-down time, an invitation to think, to examine, to meditate. In a world of driven, manic, time-compressed technology, the gift of time, Hull says, may be a considerable gift.

Remarkable Blind People

John Hull, professor of religion
Andrew Potok, artist
Eleanor Clark, writer
Helen Keller, teacher, writer
Ray Charles and Stevie Wonder, musicians
Jacques Lusseyran, French Resistance hero and Buchenwald
    survivor
Louis Braille, inventor of raised-point writing
Robert V. Hine, history professor
Historically, there were Samson, Oedipus, Homer, John Milton, among many others.

THEIR FEELINGS

The other side of courage and achievement is darkness of the spirit. There is the feeling of being seen but not seeing; of being infantilized, marginalized, the humiliation of being left out. There is a sense of the loss of status, real or imagined, at work or in the family; the sense of physical endangerment, of psychological isolation, of helplessness, worthlessness, self-hate, rage at the

16

sighted and unsighted alike.   Above all, there is the agony of being relentlessly different.

For those born blind, or blinded as babies, there is no other way to be.   Operations that have given sight after a lifetime of unsightedness have resulted in confusion. Sight is more than a sense; it is experiential and has to be learned. Oliver Sacks describes a man who was blinded as an infant through a triple illnes of meningitis, polio, and cat-scratch fever, who saw, after his operation, a confusion of light, color, shadow, a blur his brain could make no sense of. To see is not automatically to identify, and he had no idea of distance, space, or size. He had lived, as the born blind and infant blind do, in a world of touch and sound. He often closed his eyes in relief from the confused world his eyes presented until he was once more released into blindness.

It is different for those whose loss of vision is the result of later disease or trauma and disconnects a life from its most important means to information.   This loss is overwhelming, a form of psychological death, the loss of identity as a sighted person without having yet acquired an identity as a blind person.

To survive such a death and reconstruct a life takes something the world admires so much it has made the blind the darlings of the handicapped.   On the one hand, blindness is treated with the horror reserved for the castrated.   On the other, it has been elevated to the pedestal of superiority of insight and wisdom, of specialized knowledge. Perhaps it is because the tactile and auditory parts of the cerebral cortex are enhanced in compensation, or the capacity in some blind people for a kind of radar. Or perhaps it is only our own fear and a tradition of being suspicious of "otherness" that makes us treat those who are blind differently.

The worst of all our fears are heightened with the initial diagnosis of blindness:

- the fear of total dependency, of helplessness, of being treated as helpless
- the fear of rejection, loss of attractiveness, of sexuality, of constant insecurity in all relationships
- the fear of loss of work, of being treated differently, or with condescension in one's work
- the despair of depression and loneliness, isolated into an inner world, cut off from the outer one
- the feeling of shame, of being less than others
- the terror of loss or change of identity
- the sense of being unloved, and unloving

Some other possible feelings:

grief: over the loss of precious faces; the pleasures of visual beauty, of easy reading, simple unencumbered walking or running; favorite sports, watching movies; the physical freedom of quick orientation; over the loss of any object misplaced; a game that can't be played with a child, a toy found; over never knowing what new people look like; over no longer knowing what the self looks like; the loss of the spontaneous smile given and received; over no way out of the enclosing, sometimes suffocating darkness; the loss of a visual warning system for physical danger; the loss of flexibility in the imposed necessary order of the world of the blind; the loss of trees and sunsets, day and night, in many ways, of any world external to one's own body; the loss, not only of world, but of the self, faceless in any mirror.

alienation: there is sometimes the feeling of invisibility (I cannot see, therefore I cannot be seen). It is said that the illusion of privacy is a feature of the behavior of many blind adults. Hearing is sequential, touch mutual; sight is reciprocal.

anger: at the self for having the disability, at others for not; at someone else for causing it or not curing it; at the world for treating the blind as sages with the patience and fortitude of Job, or with the avoidance reserved for failure and lepers.

guilt: perhaps I am being punished for something; maybe this is my fault; I often feel I am too much of a drain on resources and time, too much trouble, an imposition on everyone around me.

low self-esteem: are my eyes disfigured? do they bulge, are they scarred by accident or surgery, do they roam, are they fixed in a stare, are they milky, closed, sunken? am I therefore ugly, or as Potok described himself, "desexed, powerless, repulsive?" am I worthless as a man or a woman, as a worker, provider, mother, father, child, friend?

fear of secondary injury or loss of another sense: an accident is always a possibility for the physically vulnerable; often the hearing blind fear most of all the loss of their hearing.

About themselves, the blind can feel fear (I can't take care of myself, no one will want to take care of me), self-doubt, worthlessness, failure (I can't see, do my work, take care of my family, compete), self-hate, rage at self, others, the universe.

19

About you, the blind can feel discomfort at your discomfort, your elaborate or misguided attempts to control and direct them, jealousy (I wish I could see, too), and personal animosity for your failure to learn about disabilities and how to respond intelligently and respectfully.

When blindness is sudden, or it is first diagnosed in someone you love, it is well to remember the stages described by Kubler-Ross when facing death: denial, anger, bargaining, depression, and acceptance. The loss of something so primary as sight is a difficult loss.

YOUR FEELINGS

About someone who is blind, or even severely visually impaired, your feelings will probably begin with feeling nervous, and uncomfortable.

Common feelings are:
I don't know what to do
I don't know why, but I'm afraid
I don't know what to say
I don't know where to look
I don't know how to act
I want to help
I don't know if my help is wanted
I don't want to make a mistake
I don't want to give offense
I don't know if your mind is affected as well as your eyes,

and if it is, how to communicate

But – I'm curious, and interested in, your blindness: how much can you see? how do you manage to live your life like that? how did you lose your sight?

And – had I better suppress or subdue my own visual responses when I'm with you?

Deeper feelings may include:

Fear: it could happen to you, too

Anxiety over possible contagion: I could get it

Relief: thankfulness it isn't you

Superiority: someone I can feel better than

Inferiority: their cross to bear is greater than mine, and they know things I don't know

Desire to avoid: I don't want to feel what I'm feeling and I don't know what to do about it

Desire to help: I have to do something

Identification: well, really, we're all human beings

Compassion: a true sorrow and affection

Caregiver syndrome: anger (at god, the doctors, the universe that it had to happen to your loved one and you); grief (at the loss of your old relationship and companionship); fear (of degeneration, of dependency); exhaustion (from doing too much of the physical and psychological work, from too much responsibity, from having to adjust, rearrange your life, your home, your schedule, your resources).

All of these feelings are less acute if someone you see or

meet or love is meeting blindness as a challenge, accepting it as a condition of life, hating it but getting on with it anyway, taking as much responsibility for life as possible.

If blindness is associated with other complicating conditions such as being very young, being very old, or other physical disabilities such as loss of hearing, or a need for a wheelchair, or prothestic limb, or is associated with brain injury or mental retardation, or complicating disease factors such as diabetes or cancer or severe and chronic depression, the feelings are more acute. This may be particularly true also if there is deformity or disfigurement, as in burn accidents.

Remind yourself:

All of us are only temporarily abled.

Almost all of us have some kind of disability, visible or invisible, of the body or the character.

Physical disability isn't the real disability in our lives. Real disability is deliberate cruelty, indifference, and the psychological death of robotic joylessnes.

3

MANNERS THAT MATTER: BOTH SIDES

Good manners are based on good will, the need to give and receive reassurance, and to share our common humanity.

But where different cultures, different worlds, different sensibilities, different abilities are concerned, good will is not enough. Good information is necessary. An excellent general rule is: *ALWAYS ASK, NEVER ASSUME.*

Good communication is circular. It is the open ability to say, with some degree of self-awareness, what you feel, need, perceive, and the sense to ask, when it is appropriate, about someone else's feelings, needs, and perceptions.

The similarities among people are obviously far greater than the dissimilarities. But there are certain emotional and experiential differences in the world of the blind that must be understood by friends on both sides of the line of sight.

You don't have to be an expert, or even understand the exact nature of an impairment. People who are blind or visually impaired are experts about themselves and their needs. Be guided by them.

THE WORLD OF THE BLIND, SOUND AND ECHO LOCATION APART, IS A WORLD OF TOUCH. AS HULL SAYS, "IT IS NOT EASY FOR SIGHTED PEOPLE TO REALIZE THE IMPLICA-

TIONS OF THE FACT THAT THE BLIND PERSON'S PERCEPTION OF THE WORLD... IS CONFINED TO THE REACH OF HIS BODY, AND TO ANY EXTENSION OF HIS BODY WHICH HE CAN SET UP, SUCH AS A CANE."

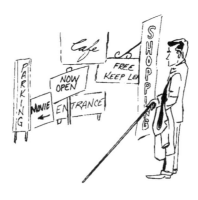

YOUR MANNERS

Don't overdo it.

There is no need to overdirect, overprotect, overcompensate, overdo. There is no need to yell, push, drag, or carry. People who have lost their sight have not necessarily lost their hearing, their minds, or control over their muscles.

People with visual impairments may seem to see better than they do. On the one hand, they may wish to explore an environment on their own to get oriented; on the other hand, they may not know someone is nearby. If you see a need and are willing help, say so. But don't take offense if your offer is declined.

Don't avoid.

A person with a disability is just another human being.

Don't grab a cane to lead, pull an arm, or ever pat or distract a seeing-eye dog on whom a blind person's life may depend. Hands, cane, dog, are all instruments of a blind person's sense perception, the way to see through touch.

Don't push when walking with someone who is blind. Let the person take your arm. The motion of your body will indicate what to do.

Don't play "guess who" games or just extend your hand in greeting. Speak your name and lightly touch the other's hand.

Don't nod, shake your head, or point when asked directions. Give clear directions, left or right, according to the way the person is facing, give numbers of buses or streets to ask for.

Don't assume a person who is blind is also ignorant or helpless, a danger in the streets to himself and others. Some have echo location, an awareness of the presence of objects and obstacles. With mobility training and a cane, the average blind person is about as safe in traffic as anyone with sight. People who are blind listen, count steps, concentrate on tactile and auditory landmarks. Too many offers of unsolicited help, too many directions (a little to the left, right, left, don't bump into the wall) can be disabling. What is helpful is to point out obstacles that aren't usually there, pick up something dropped; if you hail a cab, mention that it has arrived. Describe safety hazards; if you are walking together, don't get separated in crowds.

Don't, when visiting, move things or replace things wrong in the home. Out of place is out of the universe.for the blind.

Don't leave doors ajar, clutter on stairs or in corridors.

Don't push blind people into their chairs. Simply put a blind person's hand on the back of the chair and let her seat herself.

Don't speak to blind people through their companions, or order for them in restaurants. Talk directly, read the menu and prices. Tell him the position of the food on his plate, where her water glass is, silverware, and so forth.

Please do ask:

Ask questions about preferred methods for everything.

Ask about preferences about eating, being read to, work habits, traveling, marketing for and storing food and supplies; going to public restrooms; going out to entertainments and parties. Ask whether help is needed. Ask precisely what kind. You may not have the foggiest what is required. Be willing to be taught.

TIPS

Written materials:

Give the visually impaired person whatever cards, pamphlets, notes are going around . Help by reading, or completing forms, or by marking relevant passages for the person's usual reader.

Keep talking:

Don't fall silent when visually impaired people approach. Talking helps them orient themselves as to where people are.

And shake hands. This is also a help in placing you. Let someone who is blind know if you are leaving the room. If you begin a conversation, mention the blind person's name so he or she knows to whom you are speaking. If she is a new acquaintance, she may not mind being asked about her vision. But don't invade, don't persist, and contribute something of yourself to the conversation.

I have a friend who says, "I don't want people who are blind to have a reputation for looking frumpy. Tell me if my shoes don't match or I have on too much makeup."

Food and eating:

For the guide dog, offer to put out a dish of water.

For me, says my friend, let me know what is on my plate, where it is, where the silverware is, the water glass, and so forth, and save me from spaghetti, salads if the lettuce is not cut up, and anything generally difficult to manage. Ask if I need help -- I may be grateful.

Tips from visually impaired kids

Missy: "I want people to be aware of my eye problems so they will know why I have to use all this equipment and why I bump into people and things all the time, especially because I look like every one else. But it's not the most important thing about me.

Joe: "I never get to choose. All my teachers have me sit up front. It doesn't help, because I can't see the board anyway. The way I get notes is to give a friend carbon paper and have him make another copy for me."

Remember, people who are blind, adults and children both, have far more experience at being without sight than you do. Don't know best. Ask. Ask. Ask!

Do be willing to make mistakes. Even if you're uncomfortable, just keep trying.

Helpfulness, without heavy clouds of attention and hysteria, is a blessing.

THEIR MANNERS

Don't growl, glare, or hit with canes.

If the sighted behave offensively, remember they have not had your training, your experience, nor the mental anguish that has built or ruined your character. If they have not been physically traumatized by life, this is no reason for you to be sentenced for assault.

Don't be rude when help is offered,needed or not.

You may have been feeding yourself, laying bricks, and reading for the bar since you were six years old. But the next disabled person may have a real need for help. You don't need to insult a possible source of help for other people who are blind because you don't need it.

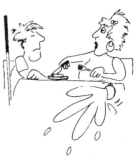

LET ME HELP

28

Be kind.

The sighted live in terror that what has happened to you could happen to them.

EDUCATE

Offer whenever you can to share information, experience, strength, and hope. Teach others that disability does not devalue someone, that ignorance, prejudice, and indifference can be the greatest problems of all. Not all people who are blind or visually impaired will work for the various Foundations, Braille Institutes, the ADA, but all can serve as role models and sources of empathy.

4

SEEKING DIAGNOSES

In Frances Neer's helpful book about living blind, *Dancing in the Dark*, her general rule for those with low vision or no vision is: make themselves known and ask for assistance. Whether they are on a bus, on the street, in a store, or in their own living rooms, they should explain themselves and ask for the help they need.

This is the most true if there is any change in someone's vision, friends, family, acquaintance, a stranger who complains in the street. Go immediately to the nearest opthalmologist for tests:

- if the eyes are red or itchy, if there is discharge
- if there is pain, or a foreign body sensation
- if there is photophobia (light hurts)
- persistant eyestrain or headache
- if vision blurs or grows cloudy, foggy, hazy
- if there is trouble with peripheral vision above, below, to the side of what you are looking at
- if there is trouble with night vision
- if there are dark or empty blind spots, specks, wrinkled effects, spots (floaters) before the eyes with flashing lights
- halos around lights

• ANY SIGNIFICANT CHANGE IN ABILITY TO SEE, ESPE-CIALLY A LESSENING OF VISION

THE AMERICAN ACADEMY OF OPTHALMOLOGY SAYS LOW VISION "IS WHEN ORDINARY EYE GLASSES OR CONTACT LENSES ARE UNABLE TO BRING A PERSON'S SIGHT UP TO NORMAL."

LEGAL BLINDNESS IS DEFINED AS VISUAL ACUITY FOR DISTANT VISION OF 20/200 OR LESS IN THE BETTER EYE WITH BEST CORRECTION.

Do not confuse:

Opthalmologist

A physician, M.D., medical doctor who treats the eye and performs eye surgery.

Optometrist

Someone trained to examine eyes, vision, and prescribe glasses. An optometrist may test for eye disease, but is not trained or certified in treatment and may not perform surgery.

Optician

A person who makes glasses.

To find an opthalmologist, call the following for recommendations:

• family physician, friends, minister, rabbi, priest, people whom you trust, for referrals

• nearest hospital, local clinic, or good university medical school

• national or local associations that serve the blind

THE EXAMINATION: RELATING TO THE DOCTOR

Doctors are trained to measure data and to draw conclusions based on scientific observation about medical issues and medical treatment. An eye doctor will ask direct questions about physical symptoms. He or she will read whatever else is necessary by examining the conjunctiva, retina, cornea, vitreous, and the functioning of other parts of the eye from lens to optic nerve.

All of this is good. There is more.

• Choose a doctor who listens carefully, who questions the clients' experience of their own symptoms and their psychological states. To ignore the client can have disastrous results on diagnoses and treatments.

• Be responsible for effective communication about problems and symptoms. Doctors may be sensitive, but they do not mind-read.

answer the questions the doctors ask: doctors know what doctors what to know

don't overload the doctor with extraneous complaints

be prepared with your information

be clear in your information and as precise and accurate as possible about symptoms

insist you understand clearly what the doctor says to you and the client; you'll be facing the "what did the doctor say" question from loved ones later on

•Be ample with your information within the confines of the appointment: this is not god or your mother and the doctor has a life, too.

32

Do understand that busy doctors often do not have the time for counseling if there is bad news. Ask the doctor for a reference to the nearest support group that serves the blind.

These are things all of us need to know about consultations with doctors. But friends of the disabled need to be doubly aware because of the greater complications involved. This is particularly true for primary caregivers.

It is true that doctors need to be as aware of their own gender,age, ethnic,religious, and any other prejudices, needs for authority, as they are of their medical facts. Some doctors, like some parents, measure their success by their patients' improvement. People must not pretend to see what they can't see on the eye chart to give their doctor a nice day!

It is true as well that clients have character defects, too. They must try to be as aware of themselves as they expect their doctor to be.

In brief, counsel your friend to:

- be clear about symptoms

- be clear about understanding the doctor's explanations

•avoid a doctor they don't like, don't trust, if it can be helped

- cooperate: the doctor can't do it alone

HEALTH-CARE SYSTEMS

Coping with the health-care system is complex enough to endanger the very sanity necessary for survival.

To be passed from one doctor to another, one facility or rehabilitation center to another, to navigate through an ocean of paper work, from doctor to insurance company, from hospital to outpatient care, to undergo the retraining or new training involved in work, the use of high-tech visual aids, Braille, mobility training, living skills training, the need for ongoing medical attention, often psychotherapy as well as physical therapy in the event of multiple trauma or defects – it's a life that could threaten the stability of an elephant.

This makes it mandatory to be persistant, to find the doctor or doctors, the therapists, the treatment centers, the rehabilitation people necessary for the life and work of a person who is blind or visually impaired.

If blindness was genetic or caused by the birth process, chances are education, rehabilitation, adaptive aids, mobility training, everything needed has been tracked from the beginning by the obstetrician, health-care system, educational system, social services systems.

If more is needed, ask for more. There are extra services for the deaf-blind, the young-blind, the elderly-blind, the blind in wheelchairs, those with multiple disabilities. Call the Board of Education and Services for the Blind in your state. Refer to the resources list at the end of this book.

5

LIVING WITH BLINDNESS: WHITE CANES AND BRAILLE

Blind people differ from each other as much as sighted people do.

JOHN HULL

Hull, university professor of religious education, explores not only what it is like to go blind, and to be blind, but the strange "other world" of blindness. "For me [the loss of sight] has been like a long, slow and lingering death... but I am more or less in control of my situation and of my work and of my feelings about it...[I have] a feeling of calmness and confidence as a blind person in a blind person's world." He reveals a world transformed, eating, lovemaking, relationships with his children, all changed, and he ends by finding in his blindness a gift.

ANDREW POTOK

Potok, a painter, wrote a portrait of an artist going blind. "The day-by-day losses of eyesight, slow and inexorable, took with them my life as a painter...my competence as a man....Going blind and passing forty, with dreams of youthful heroism and virtuosity gone forever, seemed, at times, too hard to bear." He learned to be a writer instead of a painter, and pushed on.

ELEANOR CLARK

A writer and athlete, Clark found no poetic compensations in blindness. "Who says you have to accept it, experience it, still less relish it?" But it never stopped Clark, either. Her novels, essays, memoirs, stories, and reviews flowed on. She won the National Book Award, married and mothered, traveled, and lived life to the fullest.

There are dozens of autobiographies of people who have gone blind, full of humor, courage, and ingenuity. They range from doctors to golf champions, from ballet dancers like Alison Sheen to photographers like George Covington. Writers from Homer to Milton to Helen Keller to Louis Braille, Hull, Hine, and others, have described the staggering shock and suicidal feelings of blindness. The loss of outer space, physical independence, spontaneity, the ability to drive a car, run down a street, keep pace with the rushing world, are traumatic. Even those born blind or blinded early by disease or accident talk of the frustration of living in a sighted world, often full of physical barriers and psychological prejudices.

It takes friends, family, support systems that provide services for the blind and visually impaired, courage, and the stubborness of a mule to survive.

It's the frustration of daily reality, the slow daily struggle with learning to live blind that can depress the system, dull the spirit, and make one so impatient with the stupidities of the sighted world as to make one wish the white cane were a sharpened rapier.

Patience, organization, independence, and a determination akin to whatever is possessed by high wire acrobats are the keys to the challenge of surviving blind. These, and learning major skills in a new way of living.

REHABILITATION

If treatment, medication, or surgery is indicated, don't delay. Whether blinded in an accident, or through eye disease that either now or in the future will result in visual impairment, people ought to begin rehabilitation training as soon as possible.

Living skills are best learned as soon as possible. They include:

• mobility training; cane, guide dog, the use of memory, mental maps, external cues, tactile and auditory senses; the development of sound-shadow radar for nearby objects; the use of empirical cues like sun and wind and landmarks under the feet

• Braille reading and typing

• the use of technology in communication from talking books to sound computers

• low vision aids such as closed circuit television systems to read small print,monoculars to read at a distance, Dioptic magnifiers

• the use of low tech aids from Brailled tapemeasures to Braille labelers, Brailled watches, noise-making instruments

- how to use agencies that serve the blind
- readers and visiting staff
- radio and television stations, Braille or cassette magazines, for information
- classes in the use of the telephone, counting bills and change, housekeeping, shopping, and the like

Counseling

Persuade your friend or relative to go for counseling: to help with the frustration and inconvenience of blindness, the grieving process, the feelings of being lonely, abandoned, scared, perhaps for the loss of place at work or in the family, perhaps for a sense of worthlessness, for feelings of rage.

Feelings of frustration, perhaps a resentment of too much responsibility, guilt, anger, annoyance, fear, and grief are equally normal for loved ones and friends, especially those who live with someone who is blind. Be honest about how you feel. Get help.

There are residence rehabilitation centers as well as day centers in every state.

Be in touch with:

American Foundation for the Blind
Schools for the Blind in your state
State Department for Rehabilitation
Office of Services to the Blind, State Department of
Social Services

State Department of Special Education
National Federation of the Blind

LIVING BLIND

Whether the daily techniques of living blind have been learned in a center or at home, the low vision or no vision person must now live with daily challenges to ingenuity, memory, and patience.

You will need to deal with, or help a loved one deal with:

• personal care, independent and assisted

• home organization

• communications systems from telephones to talking books to tape recorders, all assistive technology

• transportation: street, bus, escalator, and elevator travel

• public life: banks, shops, restrooms – negotiating them

• workplace: employment, education, training and retraining, vocational counseling and rehabilitation, aids and appliances, bus passes and other travel concessions (Job Opportunities for the Blind Program is operated by the National Federation of the Blind in partnership with the U.S. Department of Labor. JOB is a listing and referral service for blind job applicants)

• barriers and attitudes of the sighted – learn about the rights of the blind in the Americans with Disabilities Act, and fight for security, equality, and opportunity both in public places and in the workplace; learn about affirmative action/advocacy services

Contact your State Board of Education and Services for the Blind, or your Department of Human Resources to locate special schools. In every state, there are elementary and secondary schools for the education of those born blind or blinded young. Many states offer infant and preschool services.

In some states and communities, blind children are now mainstreamed, and, with special help, attend ordinary schools

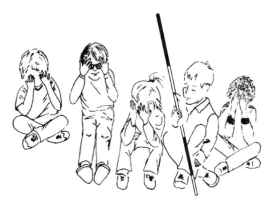

for most of the day. After the regular day, they receive specialized training in Braille and mobility skills, eventually training in a gainful occupation, as well as medical diagnosis, physical assistance, transportation, vocational guidance, and low and high tech aids instruction.

In what Potok calls the extensive blind empire, there is controversy over the advantages and disadvantages of mainstreaming. On the good side, it teaches children early on that being blind is just another human condition. On the down side, blind children may receive less of the specialized training in Braille, the use of the white cane, and other specialized living skills than they need.

MULTIPLE DISABILITIES

There are those for whom blindness is only part of the battle to survive life. There are the very young blind, trying to learn to crawl without injury, find food and find their mouths to put it in. There are the elderly blind, trying to find any meaning in their lives at all. There are the deaf-blind, who deal simultaneously with two disabilities, cut off both from sight and sound. Helen Keller proved it could be done, with a lot of courage and a lot of help. There are the people who are blind and because of disease or accident are confined to wheelchairs as well as darkness.

I have a friend whose daughter is blind and who lives in a wheelchair who says she never gets used to being confined to one space and to darkness. She says she feels suffocated, panicked by being nearly helpless, as if she were living in a tomb. She says it cheerfully, but she means it. And then she goes back to the clients on her counseling schedule. She has her Master's degree in Social Work.

She says, "Tell people that disability is a technicality. It doesn't have to be a way of life."

41

6

RESOURCES: TECHNIQUES AND ASSISTIVE AIDS; COMMUNICATION AIDS; MOBILITY AIDS; COSMETIC EYES; RETRAINING; NEW TRAINING; THE WORKPLACE AND ADA; FUNDS

Most people who are blind manage very well. They manage far better in many ways than sighted people think.

Whether born blind, struck blind by accident or an operation for retinal cancer, or enduring the slow process of diminishing sight from glaucoma, retinitis pigmentosa, or macular degeneration, everyone with impaired vision can benefit from the quite extraordinary resources, services, and organizations of the blind and for the blind.

Everyone benefits particularly from learning about techniques, adaptive aids, and assistive devices as early as possible.

INDEPENDENT LIVING SKILLS

Order, organization, the development of memory skills, and experimenting with what works best for the individual; these are the main things.

Order and organization

Help your friend to organize and remember where things that are used and needed belong, and to tell everyone not to use anything without replacing it exactly where it is supposed to be. For someone who can't see, gone is gone!

Markers – tape, rubber bands, Braille or ordinary letter labelers, devices like special bags for storage – all will give you appropriate information for what your closets and drawers contain. Helpful gadgets can be ordered from catalogs, and by visiting stores that sell equipment for the blind. You can call Lighthouse Low Vision Products at 1-800-453-4923.

Pay particular attention to order in the areas of the home – kitchen, bathroom, home office, closet – that mean the most.

There are many systems, tricks, methods to use.

Some people hang all parts of an outfit together in separate closet bags, for instance. Some buy socks all the same color. There can be hangers for same-color ties, separate drawer bags for bras and pantyhose. There can be separate boxes on a desk for incoming and outgoing mail awaiting reader or secretarial assistance, drawers labeled for checkbooks, manuscripts, Braille paper and tools. Labelers are helpful for carpenter benches and tool boxes, for sewing and knitting supplies, especially to sort out colors.

With constant touching and keeping track of things, insistance on others not scrambling personal effects, patience at the slow time some things take, chaos can be systematized into manageable order.

Gadgets

One friend who is blind prefers battery-operated gadgets to electrical appliances. She says this avoids the risk of shock, wire

43

confusion, crawling around for outlets, and tripping over cords in both kitchen and office.

Talking clocks (when was the toast in?), automatic microwave ovens (was the the burner still on?) are good kitchen controls.

"Memo pad" tape recorders, radios, telephones in as many rooms as possible save time and movement. Scissors and knives in safe places, closed cabinet and room doors, uncluttered floors and stairs save accidents.

In the bathroom, carpeting, non-skid tiles, non-skid rubber bath mats, handrails and grab bars, even a walker in the shower,these and caution (stepping into too hot a tub, an uncovered razor, the wrong medicine bottle) – all these are useful inhibitors.

Attend some classes in independent living skills for training and more suggestions for home management and office with your friend.

COMMUNICATIONS

Insist that your friend learn some Braille.

•	:	••	•:	•.	:•	::
A	B	C	D	E	F	G
:.	•'	.:	:	:	••	::
H	I	J	K	L	M	N
:•	:•	::	:•	:•	::	..
O	P	Q	R	S	T	U
:.	•:	::	::	.:		
V	W	X	Y	Z		

It may be a slower process than sight reading, but no information will be inaccessible if the blind can read books, magazines, manuals, and everything Braille-labeled from elevator floors to raised maps on their own. There are Braille hand tools, Braille typewriters, and computer keyboards, Brailled scientific instruments, music, knobs for appliances, telephones, remotes, services that create custom-made aids for most conceivable vision disability needs.

As has been mentioned, for mainstreamed children in primary and secondary schools, or among people who are blinded later in life, Braille may remain awkward, less practiced. Recordings for the blind, talking books (large print books and low vision aids), sound computers and other computer hardware, cassette players, and an astonishing array of optical aids, high technology devices to meet the needs of people who are blind and deaf-blind are available.

Call The Sensory Access Foundation (415-329-0430), Innovative Rehabilitation Technology, Inc. (415-961-3161), Smith-Kettlewell Institute of Visual Sciences Rehabilitation Engineering Services (415-561-1620), Telesensory Systems, Inc. (415-960-0920) for special communications needs. Assistive technology is available.

For listening to the world, contact:

In Touch: Satellite Radio, Radio Broadcast for the Blind Program, 15 West 65th Street, New York, N.Y. 10023. It is a radio station that is on 24 hours a day, 7 days a week. Special receivers are needed to hear these radio programs.

TV: Descriptive Video Service for the visually impaired. Contact your local public television station.

Telephone: Call the business office for **FREE** services for the blind.

Public Library/Communications Center: Your local library has talking books on cassette tapes and records, cassette and record players to borrow, and a bibliography of book and magazine titles on tape or soft disc recording -- all FREE to borrow.

Choice Magazine Listening, 85 Channel Drive, Port Washington, NY 11050. National magazines on cassette tapes FREE of charge.

Recordings for the Blind. Scholarly library. Check local telephone book.

The Lighthouse. Adult activities, information, and classes. Check local telephone book.

JUST ORDINARY COMMUNICATION

On the subject of just ordinary communication between people, the only thing that makes people who are blind different from anyone else is that they cannot see.

Some people who are blind may want to touch your hand or

46

your face or your shoulder to discover your features, your height, the shape of your presence as they might a sculpture or a flower. Some may not. You've noticed it is the same with sighted people. Some are touchers, some are not.

I have one friend who is blind who rejects the business of touching people he does not know well altogether. He is terrified a hairpiece or an eyelash will come off in his hand.

Sighted people are often curious about sex among blind people. It is sad not to see the person you are making love to, but making love is mostly about touching bodies, experiencing union, and feeling good. In bed, we are the same in these matters, equal, the sighted and the not. I am informed that the occasional kiss misses the mark. But from Milton to Helen Keller, most blind people have had love lives.

MOBILITY AIDS

What is available are white canes and guide dogs.
Canes
Canes come in different lengths. For most adults, they are 5 feet or 6 feet long, but they may be cut down to any length that is comfortable. A mobility trainer or simple experience will indicate what length is needed. Canes for the blind are white, red-tipped, straight-handled like a staff, with a wrist strap.

They come in different materials. I know a mountain climber who is blind for whom the wood ones last only a couple of hours. He prefers aluminum. Most are made of fiber glass.

They come in ordinary form or laser form. The laser cane senses objects at five feet, and lets the user know through a series of vibrations what is near. Canes can be straight, or collapsible, folding up easily for walking with a sighted friend or riding on a crowded bus.

By tapping or moving the cane low in a three-foot arc, obstacles can be felt in front of the feet.

White canes are used not only for mobility, but to attract the attention of others so they know to watch out for a blind person. Especially in crossing streets, the cane should be held slightly lifted and moving. This protective device attracts the notice of drivers and pedestrians.

Guide Dogs

The Seeing Eye is one organization that trains guide dogs for blind people. Ask for the guide dog service in your city or state.

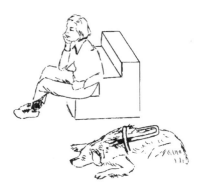

Seeing Eye pups are especially raised, numbered, and obedience-trained. They are mostly German shepherds, Labrador retrievers, golden retrievers, and generally females. Females are gentler, less aggressive, less easily distracted. Guide dogs are working dogs, must be in top physical condition, and must learn never to be distracted by strange people or strange surroundings, not to bark or growl, frighten people, or to make a nuisance of themselves.

They are trained in lightweight, leather-covered harnesses with body strap, collar, and leash. A new owner is trained as thoroughly as the dog, in pace, commands, physical signals, obedience techniques, praise, and care. There are federal regulations that permit any blind person to be accompanied by a guide dog in passenger sections of public transportation and in public buildings.

COSMETIC EYES

Prosthetic eyes are usually made of special plastic. They look real, and only need to be taken out every week or two and cleaned.

RETRAINING; NEW TRAINING;
THE WORKPLACE AND ADA (Americans with Disabilities Act)

The State Department of Rehabilitation offers services that include instruction in Braille, typing, homemaking, daily living skills, and independent travel. The vocational rehabilitation program offers job preparation services, training and retraining, vocational counseling and evaluation, medical consultations, job placement.

Also call:

The National Federation of the Blind

Office of Services to the Blind, State Department of
Social Services

Veterans Administration, Rehabilitation Center

American Foundation for the Blind

JOB: Job Opportunities for the Blind

This organization is a listing and referral service for blind job applicants, provides special material to deaf-blind applicants in Braille, distributes recorded form materials, receives from employers listings of vacant positions throughout the country, and conducts not only seminars for blind and deaf-blind applicants to help them learn about their rights, about laws and regulations pertaining to employment of the blind, but holds workshops for employers.

All these organizations offer resources for retraining and new training in old or new, vocational and occupational work.

Problems with training and retraining will be fewer than getting bosses to accept the services of people who are blind or who have impaired vision. But it is time for the United States to recognize the blind as a competent and energetic minority capable of holding a wide variety of positions in fields as various as administration, sales, banking, counseling, pharmacology, social work, teaching, electrical engineering, medicine, the law, and almost everything else.

People with disabilities are just that: they are people. And they would rather be working and living in the mainstream than isolated and dependent on welfare.

ADA

The Americans with Disabilities Act prohibits discrimination in the workplace. It describes and prohibits the persistant discrimination experienced by people with disabilities in:

- employment
- housing
- public accommodations
- education
- transportation, communication, recreation
- health services, access to public services, voting
- outright, intentional exclusion, segregation or relegation to lesser programs
- architectural, transportation, communication barriers
- included also are people for whom public prejudice may constitute a disability: those with HIV virus; people with facial disfigurement that is disabling only because of the attitudes and reactions of others (people blinded and scarred in fires and explosions often run into this)

But while there are many resources, organizations, and services, schools and technologies, myths and old attitudes persist. The ADA's insistance on reasonable accommodation is not enough. Education is necessary.

It begins with mainstreaming children with disabilities so that all children accept each other as differently abled, not as different.

It ends with adults understanding we are all only temporarily abled, and that our energies are far better employed concentrating on the abilities rather than disabilities in all of us.

FUNDS

Any disability can be expensive, from special schooling to special assistive technology.

For funding, contact your State Department of Social Services(phone numbers in the government section of any telephone book), Board of Education and Services for the Blind, your local chapter of the National Federation of the Blind for appropriate assistance and advice.

There is public assistance for people with disabilities, medical assistance instead of insurance. There are sources for independent living with an attendant, group homes, rehabilitation centers, education, and training. A list of some of these resources has been added at the end of the book.

In particular, the National Federation of the Blind, the largest organization of the blind in America, has as its purpose the complete integration of the blind into society on a basis of equality, and the removal of legal, economic, and social discrimination. NFB is the blind speaking for themselves, advocating for themselves, and providing a forum for blinded persons to share experiences, techniques, and opportunities.

7
AT HOME AND OUT THERE

Behave in public as you would in private with a friend who is blind. When you are out in the community, shopping, at theater, eating in a restaurant, your behavior will teach others both about what the ADA means by "reasonable accommodation" and what you understand are appropriate courtesies. Often our behavior with our friends who are blind changes and opens attitudes as much as technology, training, and the law changes and opens opportunities.

SOURCES FOR HELP

It is important for people who are blind and for people who care about them to join local and national associations for the blind and of the blind. This not only helps blind people to achieve all they can, but to exercise to the fullest their individual talents and capacities, their right to work along with sighted people in all professions, skilled trades, occupations.

These association can provide lists of support groups, literature, recordings, talking books, magazines, medical journal articles. To support these associations and organizations also helps to support research and expand services.

National Federation of the Blind, 1800 Johnson Street, Baltimore, Maryland 21230. (301) 659-9314, or call your state office.

American Foundation for the Blind, 15 West 16th Street, New York, N.Y. 10011. (800) 232-5463.

Association for Education and Rehabilitation of the Blind and Visually Impaired, 206 North Washington St., Suite 320, Alexandria, VA 22314. (703) 548-1884.

American Council of the Blind, 1155 15th Street, N.W., Suite 720, Washington, D.C. 20005. (800) 424-8666. This organization acts as a national clearinghouse for information, publishes "The Braille Forum," and provides legal assistance, scholarships.

American Printing House for the Blind, PO Box 6085, Louisville, KY 40206. (800)223-1839.

Recording for the Blind, 20 Roszel Road, Princeton, NJ 08540. (609)452-0606.

National Organization on Disability, 910 16th Street, N.W., Washington, DC 20006. (800) 248-ABLE.

Rehabilitation Services Administration, U.S. Department of Education, 330 C Street, S.W. Washington, DC 20001. (202) 732-1282.

National Council on Disability, 800 Independence Avenue, S.W., Suite 814, Washington, DC 20591. (202) 267-3235.

The above organizations will inform you of local organzations and specialized organizations such as for sports, or the arts, or for multiple disability or multi-sensory support groups.

Also:

State Department of Rehabilitation

Office of Services to the Blind, State Department of Social Services Veteran's Administration, Rehabilitation Center

State Department of Education, Schools for the Blind

There are:

Arts and disability organizations:

Very Special Arts, an educational affiliate of the John F. Kennedy

Center for the Performing Arts, (800) 933-8721.

Athletic organizations, international, national, and local sports associations, with teaching clinics and competitive events, and junior divisions.

For high and low assistive technology, some resources have already been listed.

Check your Yellow Pages for your nearest Lighthouse number for more information. Or write to: Lighthouse Low Vision Products, 36-20 Northern Blvd., Long Island City, N.Y. 11101. (800) 453-4923.

For other catalogues and magazines:

Resources for Rehabilitation, 33 Bedford Street, Suite 19A, Lexington, MA 02173. (617) 862-6455.

LANTERN, The Lighthouse

Do not forget to consult your doctor, your opthalmologist, your community-assistance organizations, and medical health-care professionals.

SELECTED REFERENCE BIBLIOGRAPHY

Coombs, Jan, *Living with the Disabled: You Can Help,* New York, Sterling Pub. Co., Inc., 1984.

Hine, Robert V., *Second Sight,* Berkeley, Los Angeles, London,Univ. California Press, 1993.

Hull, John M. Hull, *Touching the Rock, An Experience of Blindness,* New York, Pantheon, 1990.

Kettelkamp, Larry, *High Tech for the Handicapped,* Hillside, N.J., Enslow Publishers, Inc., 1991.

Krementz, Jill, *How It Feels to Live with a Physical Handicap,* New York, Simon & Schuster, 1992.

Neer, Frances Lief, *Dancing in the Dark,* San Francisco, Rebecca House, 1994.

Potok, Andrew, *Ordinary Daylight, Portrait of an Artist Going Blind,* New York, Holt, Rinehart and Winston, 1980.

Rosenberg, Michael S., Ph.D., and Irene Edmond-Rosenberg, M.P.A.,*The Special Education Sourcebook, A Teacher's Guide to Programs, Materials, and Information Sources,* Woodbine House, 1994.

Sacks, Oliver, M.D., *An Anthropologist on Mars, "To See and Not See,"* New York, Knopf, 1995.

Smith, Jean Kennedy (founder of Very Special Arts), and George Plimpton, *Chronicles of Courage,* New York, Random House, 1993.

Tierney, Lawrence M., Jr., M.D., Stephen J. McPhee, M.D., and Maxine A. Papadakis, M.D., *Current Medical Diagnosis & Treatment,* Norwalk, CT, Appleton & Lange, 1995.

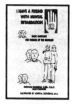
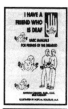

BICK
PUBLISHING HOUSE
PRESENTS
WIND OVER WINGS PRESS

BASIC MANUAL
WILDLIFE REHABILITATION SERIES
IN 6 VOLUMES

I FOUND A BABY BIRD
ISBN: 1-884158-00-5
Volume 1
Price: $6.25

I FOUND A BABY RABBIT
ISBN: 1-884158-03-x
Volume 4
Price $6.25

I FOUND A BABY SQUIRREL
ISBN: 1-884158-01-3
Volume 2
Price $6.25

I FOUND A BABY OPOSSUM
ISBN: 1-884158-06-4
Volume 5
Price $6.25

I FOUND A BABY DUCK
ISBN: 1-884158-02-1
Volume 3
Price $6.25

I FOUND A BABY RACCOON
ISBN: 1-884158-05-6
Volume 6
Price $6.25

- For parents, teachers, librarians who want to learn and teach basic rehabilitation
- For backyard rehabilitators
- For rehabilitation centers, to sell to volunteers

Order from your local bookstore through:
BAKER & TAYLOR
INLAND BOOK COMPANY

or by writing or calling:
WILDLIFE REHABILITATION TODAY MAGAZINE
Coconut Creek Publishing Co.
2201 NW 40TH Terrace
Coconut Creek, FL 33066
(305) 972-6092   ■ Perfect bound editions available ■